Diabetes Cooking

93 Diabetes Recipes for Breakfast Lunch Dinner Snacks and Smoothies A Guide to Diabetes Foods to Help You Prepare Healthy Delicious Diabetes Meals for Total Diabetes Control

By John McArthur

Copyright

ISBN-13:978-1495914225
ISBN-10:1495914224

Natural Health Magazine

www.naturalhealthmagazine.net

The information in this book is provided for educational and information purposes only. It is not intended to be used as medical advice or as a substitute for treatment by a doctor or healthcare provider.

The information and opinions contained in this publication are believed to be accurate based on the information available to the author. However, the contents have not been evaluated by the U.S. Food and Drug Administration and are not intended to diagnose, treat, cure or prevent disease.

The author and publisher are not responsible for the use, effectiveness or safety of any procedure or treatment mentioned

Warning

All treatment of any medical condition (without exception) must always be done under supervision of a qualified medical professional. The fact that a substance is "natural" does not necessarily mean that it has no side effects or interaction with other medications.

Medical professionals are qualified and experienced to give advice on side effects and interactions of all types of medication.

Table of Contents

Foreword

It is a scientific fact that diabetics can control their condition effectively with the right diet, natural supplements and herbs. With a few lifestyle changes they can live a normal and healthy life.

A low-fat, high-fiber, whole-food diet packed with vegetables, fruits, nuts, seeds and lean protein is encouraged.

The advice in this book will give you a good understanding of diabetes and includes more than 90 recipes to help you prepare delicious meals, snacks and smoothies.

Diabetics don't have to settle for monotonous bland and unimaginative food. You will see that there are many ways to prepare healthy and delicious meals.

The Diabetes Diet Solution

Introduction

If you are reading this book you most likely know someone who suffers from diabetes or you have been diagnosed with the condition. The incidence of diabetes is rising at an alarming rate and this can largely be attributed to the way our diet has changed over the years. The health of thousands of people around the world is being crippled by diabetes as unhealthy diet choices become the norm in our households.

As you may know, diabetes is characterized by abnormal levels of sugar and glucose in the blood. Type I Diabetes, also known as Juvenile onset diabetes, accounts for only 10% of all cases. Type II Diabetes affects as much as 90% of all diabetic suffers and although the onset can partially be blamed on genetics in some cases, most of the time it is causes by being overweight, lack of exercise, high blood pressure, obesity and poor diet choices. Type II Diabetics struggle with raised glucose levels in their blood which is a result of the loss of sensitivity to insulin by the cells of the body. The goal in the treatment of both Type I and Type II diabetes is to ensure that blood sugar levels remain normal. For those with Type II diabetes, the best and most effective way of doing this is by making changes to their diet. I hope to give you dietary guidelines and delicious recipes that will make managing your condition much easier than you ever imagined. At the end of the day, diet and nutrition play a crucial role in the treatment and prevention of diabetes, especially type II diabetes. Learning to make healthy food choices will help you to ensure normal blood sugar levels are maintained and will either eliminate certain symptoms or at least keep them under control.

Basic Diabetic Dietary Guidelines

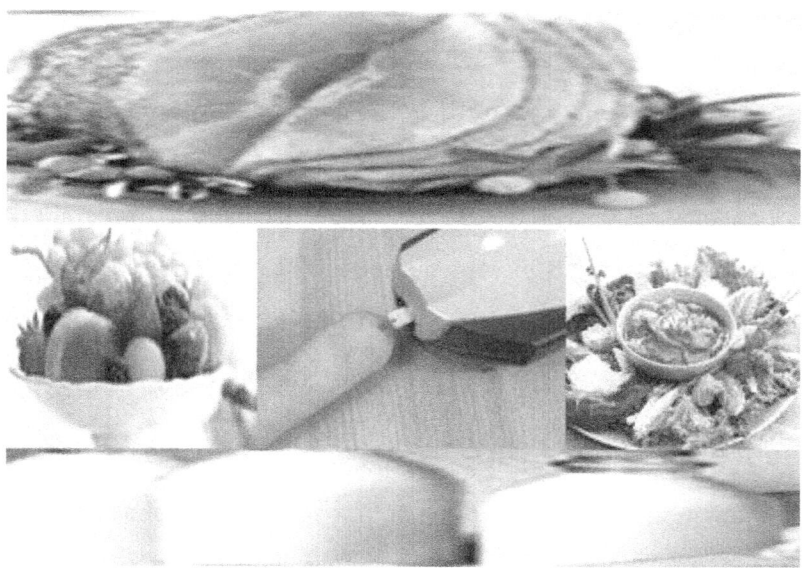

It's All About Balance

I'm sure that at some point in your life you have had someone tell you that it is important to eat a balanced diet. Although this guideline is applicable to everyone, it is especially important and highly beneficial to diabetics. Diabetics should aim to eat meals that have a good balance of fats, proteins and carbohydrates. This is easier to achieve than it seems since most snacks and meals naturally contain these components. The goal should be to make sure you are eating a variety of items from the recommended food groups in the right amounts. Later on I will show you easy, affordable ways to practically make that happen.

Say No To Excess Calories

If you are a diabetic – type 2 in particular - it is crucial that you remain mindful of what you are eating. How much sugar, saturated fat, and fat is in your diet and is there any way it can reduced if it is excessive? Diabetics who don't keep their weight down often struggle with circulatory issues and other sicknesses. This can so easily be avoided if enough attention is given to diet. It is important to remember that reducing sugar and fat in your diet does not mean that it needs to be completely eliminated. You just need to have certain measures in place to help you control and monitor your calorie intake.

Reduce Fats And Sugars

The thought of completely cutting out fat and sugar is usually too terrible for anyone to contemplate. The good news is that there are many ways for diabetics to make changes that don't always involve the complete elimination of the things they used to eat. Here are some practical ways to help you reduce the amount of fat and sugar in your diet.

- As a rule avoid all sweets and chocolate bars since they are extremely high in calories and always cause an instant spike in blood sugar. The only exception is if a sweet or chocolate bar is eaten before or after a period of prolonged physical activity. One option is to try and buy chocolate in very thin tablets or maybe as drops and to eat only one block or drop at a time. It usually only takes a small amount to satisfy a sugar craving.

- Always pay attention to labels to find out if there is added sugar in the items you are buying. One example is canned fruit which is canned in either syrup or fruit juice. Obviously the fruit canned in fruit juice would be the better option, although this would also need to be eaten in moderation. Remember that sugar has many other names such as lactose, malt, glucose, sucrose, fructose, honey, corn syrup etc. It is important for diabetics to become familiar with these terms so that they are well equipped to monitor their sugar intake.

- If baking was your thing before being diagnosed with diabetes that certainly does not need to change. Instead of using sugar you can rather use fresh or dried fruits. Fruit naturally has fructose, but your body will absorb this slowly unlike granulated sugar.

- All fizzy sugary drinks should be avoided. Try drinking fresh fruit juice or fizzy water instead. If you really want a soda from time to time then opt for one that is artificially sweetened and low in calories.

- One important change that diabetics will need to make is the elimination of sugar in their tea and coffee. It is ideal to completely stop sweetening these drinks but if it is really tough artificial sweeteners are the better option.

The Diabetic's Shopping List

I am going to give you a comprehensive list of foods in different categories so that you will know what foods you can eat and what foods should be avoided as far as possible. Unfortunately it isn't really black and white as there are many foods which are considered "borderline." They don't need to be completely avoided, but it is important to eat these foods in the correct quantities and to make sure you never overindulge. I will also give you a list of foods that are considered "free foods." These foods can be eaten at any time and in any quantity.

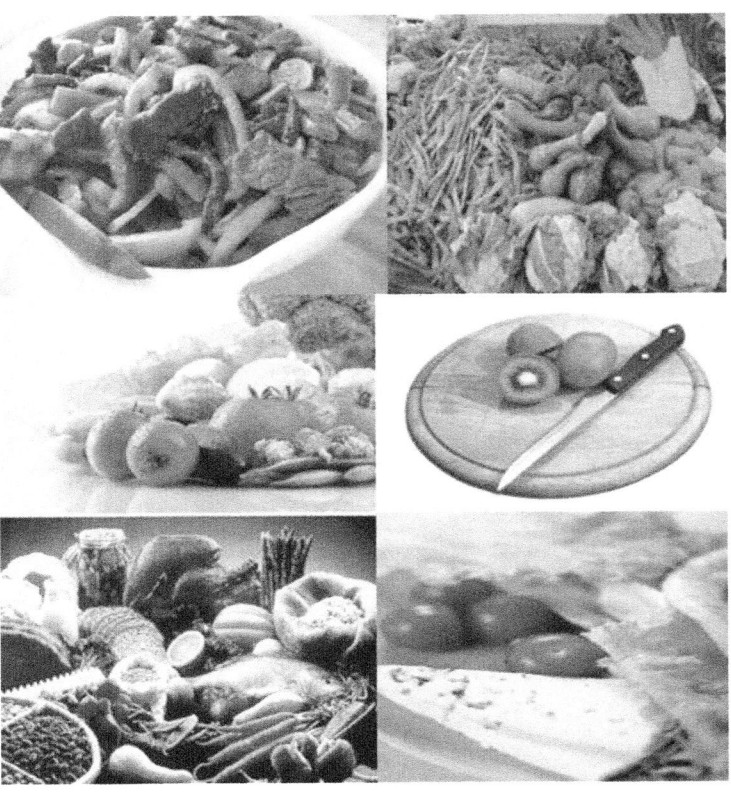

Good Foods

The following list contains foods which are considered good for diabetics. These proteins and carbohydrates should be part of your daily allocation of foods and should not exceed your daily limit.

- Meat products and lean meats
- All peas, beans and pulses
- Whole-wheat pasta and brown rice
- All fresh fruits
- All root vegetables
- Wholemeal flours, breads, oats, and biscuits (unsweetened)
- Canned fruits that have been canned in fruit juice, not syrup
- Dried fruit
- Unsweetened high-fibre cereals
- Fish (Fresh or frozen)
- Skimmed milk
- Low fat cheese and yoghurts
- All Soya products

Borderline Foods

These foods are not considered to be good carbohydrates and proteins but can be eaten in moderation from time to time.

- Jams, marmalades and spreads that have reduced sugar
- Bread, white flour, rice, pasta, pastry, unsweetened biscuits
- Semolina, arrowroot, cornflour
- Potato products that have been fried (eg. Potato Chips)

- Sausages and other fatty meats

- Fish products and salty meats

- Fruit juice

- Alcohol

- Breakfast cereals (unsweetened)

- Full cream milk, cheese, cream and yoghurt

Bad Foods

The following list contains foods that should really be avoided at all cost. They are not beneficial to diabetics at all. If they are consumed occasionally, they must be eaten in extremely small quantities.

- Ice-cream, sweets, candy, ice lollies etc.

- Caster, granulated, and Demerara sugar as well as honey and golden syrup

- Full sugar chewing gum

- Full sugar spreads, marmalades and jams

- Cakes, biscuits, and buns made from sugar and white flour

- All desserts that have been made with refined sugar and flour

- Sugary breakfast cereals

- Canned fruit in syrup

- Sugary fizzy drinks, sodas, and fruit squash

Free Foods

If you are ever in the mood to over indulge you can pick a food from the following list. These foods are considered free – you can eat and enjoy them to your heart's content since they are very low in fat, sugar and calories.

- Onions (all different types)
- All leafy and green vegetables
- All cruciferous vegetables (broccoli, turnip, cabbage and cauliflower)
- Salad vegetables like cucumbers, tomatoes, peppers etc;)
- Green beans and peas
- Mushrooms
- Berries like redcurrants, cranberries and loganberries
- Coffee, tea, and water
- Clear soups
- Tomato juice

Breakfast Recipes

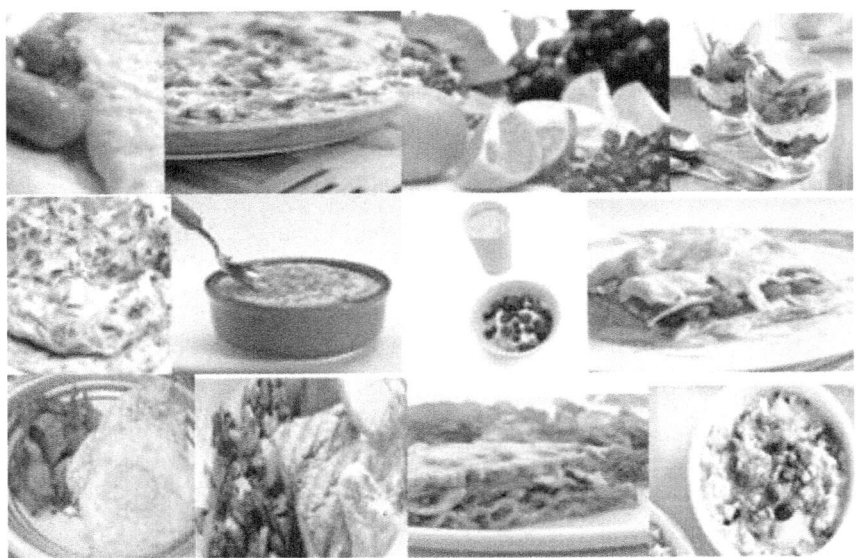

English Muffin Topped With Sausage Tomato And Cheese

Ingredients

1 whole grain English muffin

1 turkey or vegetable sausage patty

1 slice reduced fat cheese

Preparation

- Toast the English muffin and heat your sausage at the same time.
- Place the heated sausage onto your muffin and top with the slice of cheese. It's that easy!

Whole Wheat Cranberry Scones

Ingredients

½ cup whole wheat flour

1 ½ cups all-purpose flour

2 ¼ tsp Stevia powdered extract (18 -27 drops Stevia liquid concentrate)

¼ tsp baking soda

1 tsp cinnamon

1 ½ tsp baking powder

¼ tsp salt

1/3 cup butter

½ cup egg substitute

1/3 cup buttermilk

1 cup dried cranberries

3 tbsp rolled oats

Preparation

- Preheat your oven to 392 deg. F (200 deg. Celsius).
- In a large mixing bowl combine all the dry ingredients and blend thoroughly. Crumble the butter into the dry mixture and then make

a hole in the middle of the mixture as you push it onto the sides of the bowl.

- In a separate mixing bowl combine the buttermilk, eggs and cranberries and then pour this mixture into the center of the dry mixture. Stir until combined.

- On a flat floured surface, knead the dough and then spread it out so that it is 8 inches wide and about ¾ inch thick. Brush buttermilk onto the top and sprinkle the oats over and push them into the dough.

- Divide the dough to make 12 separate scones and then place them onto a baking sheet (must not be greased).

- Bake in the oven for about 15 minutes until golden brown.

Cheese And Asparagus Omelet

Ingredients

½ cup egg substitute

4 spears of asparagus

Non-stick cooking spray

½ tsp olive oil

¼ tsp ground black pepper

1 fat-free or low fat cheese wedge cut into pieces

1 tbsp sweet red peppers

1 tsp chopped parsley

Preparation

- Lightly coat an unheated large non-stick skillet with cooking spray. Add asparagus to skillet and pan-roast over medium-high heat for 7 minutes or until browned and tender, turning occasionally. Set aside.
- In a medium bowl combine egg whites and pepper. Using a fork, beat until combined but not frothy. In an 8-inch non-stick skillet heat oil over medium-high heat. Add egg whites to skillet. Reduce heat to medium. As eggs start to set, use a heatproof silicone spatula to gently lift edges of set egg white, tilting pan to allow liquid egg white to run under set egg. Continue until egg is set but still shiny.

- Arrange the asparagus spears on half of the eggs in skillet. Top evenly with cheese. Fold the unfilled half of the eggs over the asparagus and cheese. Gently slide the omelet out of the skillet onto a serving plate. Sprinkle omelet with red sweet pepper slivers and parsley. Makes 1 omelet serving.

Omelet With A Spanish Twist

Ingredients

3 beaten eggs

1 tsp olive oil

1 chopped red onion

1 chopped green pepper

1/2 cup peeled chopped potatoes

1 tbsp chopped parsley

1 tbsp parmesan cheese

Salt and pepper

Preparation

- In a medium sized pot boil the potatoes until they are soft.
- In a separate pan fry the onions and peppers in the tsp of olive oil for a few minutes.
- Add the cooked potato and parsley to the fried onions and peppers and combine.
- In a separate bowl combine the beaten eggs with the parmesan.
- Pour the egg mixture over the contents in the pan and cook for around 3 minutes.
- To finish off place the pan under a hot grill until the omelet has turned golden brown.

Whole Wheat Bagel With Peanut Butter And Banana

Ingredients

1 Whole wheat Bagel

1 tbsp peanut butter

1 thinly sliced banana

Preparation

- Slice the bagel in half and spread the peanut butter onto both sides.
- Evenly distribute the banana slices.
- Close the bagel and enjoy a quick healthy breakfast!

Pita Pocket With Cottage Cheese And Walnuts

Ingredients

1 whole grain pita pocket

½ cup low fat cottage cheese

½ cup chopped walnuts

Preparation

- Combine the low fat cottage cheese and walnuts
- Spoon the mixture into your pita pocket and enjoy.

Guilt-Free Breakfast Pizza

Ingredients

1 whole wheat thin pizza base

¼ cup cheese

2 tbsp pizza sauce

1 tbsp of chopped green pepper

1 tbsp fresh basil

Preparation

- Spread the pizza sauce on the base and then add the basil, cheese, green pepper, and basil.
- Place in the microwave for 1 min until the cheese has melted.

Crispy Hotcakes Topped With Yoghurt And Blueberries

Ingredients

1 3/4 cup self-raising flour (wholemeal)

1 cup fresh blueberries

3 cups fat free yoghurt

1/2 cup apple sauce

1 tsp vanilla extract

1 separated egg

Egg whites from 2 eggs

Preparation

- Beat the egg whites together until you see soft peaks have formed.
- In a medium sized bowl combine the flour, 1/2 of the blueberries, vanilla extract, apple sauce, and 2 cups of the yoghurt. Once properly combined, fold in the egg whites.
- Heat oil in a frying pan and use 1/4 cup of the batter for one hotcake. When frying, only turn once bubbles have started forming on the surface. They should be golden brown and cooked through.
- Once cooked, top each hotcake with some of the remaining blueberries and yogurt. (Serves 6)

Delicious Oats Filled With Bananas And Walnuts

Ingredients

1 1/3 cup rolled oats

2 cups water

1 cup low-fat milk

2 thickly sliced medium sized bananas

1/2 cup chopped walnuts

1 tbsp honey

1 additional cup low-fat milk (for use on cooked oats – optional)

Preparation

- Pour the water and the milk (1 cup) into a pot and bring to the boil.
- Lower the heat and add oats. Allow to simmer for about 5 min. Oats should be soft and creamy when ready.
- Put oats in bowls and top with honey, walnuts and banana sliced. Add extra milk if desired. (Serves 4)

Rye Bread With Poached Eggs And Salmon

Ingredients

4 large eggs

4 slices of toasted rye bread

7 oz. smoked salmon

6 oz. halved asparagus strips

Salt and pepper to taste

Preparation

- To poach eggs, fill a medium sized pan with water (only half way) and bring to the boil. Break each egg into a cup (separately) and gently pour into water. Once the 4 eggs are in the water allow water to start boiling again.\
- Once water has started boiling, turn down heat and allow eggs to cook for around 4 minutes.
- Gently remove each egg and place on a paper towel to soak up water.
- Cook Asparagus by steaming or boiling.
- Place rye break on plates and stack salmon and asparagus, and then egg on top. Sprinkle salt and pepper over the top if desired.

Fluffy Blueberry Muffins

Ingredients

2 cups self-raising flour – one white and the other wholemeal

1 Tbsp Stevia powdered extract (1 tsp Stevia liquid concentrate)

2 beaten egg whites

1/3 cup apple sauce

3/4 cup low-fat milk

150g blueberries

Preparation

- Grease a muffin pan that is big enough to make 12 muffins and preheat oven to 356 deg. F (180 deg. Celsius).
- Sift flour (both types) into a large bowl and then add Stevia.
- In a separate small bowl combine the milk, apple sauce and egg whites. Once combined pour wet mixture into dry mixture and finish off by stirring in the blueberries.
- Spoon the mixture into the 12 separate muffin holes before placing in oven and baking for around 20 minutes.

Rye Bread Topped With Corn, Ricotta And Spinach

Ingredients

1 can corn kernels (drained)

1/2 cup chopped spinach leaves

2 tbsp low-fat ricotta cheese

1 slices toasted rye bread

Preparation

- Place drained corn in microwaveable bowl and heat on high for 30 seconds.
- Stir ricotta cheese and spinach into corn.
- Place rye bread on plate and top each slice with the corn, cheese and spinach combination.

Wholesome Homemade Berry Muesli

Ingredients

1 cup rolled oats

1/2 cup all-bran

1/4 cup dried cranberries

2 cups low-fat milk

1 sliced large banana

1/2 cup juicy fresh raspberries

Preparation

- Mix the rolled oats, all bran and cranberries to make your muesli.
- Place muesli in bowls and finish off by topping with raspberries, milk and banana slices. Guaranteed to be crispy and delicious!

Scrambled Eggs The Spanish Way

Ingredients

Cooking spray

3 large eggs

1 1/2 cups egg substitute

3/4 cup finely chopped tomatoes

1/4 cup finely chopped green bell peppers

1/4 cup shredded green onions

1/4 cup fat-free milk

1/4 tsp salt

1/4 tsp black pepper teaspoon black pepper

1/8 tsp hot sauce

Preparation

- Heat oil in a large pan and then fry tomatoes, bell peppers and onions. Once that is done remove from heat and set aside.
- In a bowl combine the egg, egg substitute, milk, salt, pepper and hot sauce and mix well with a whisk.
- Pour the mixture into the pan and cook on low heat. Stir every now and then and remove once eggs are cooked.

- Stir the fried tomato, bell pepper and onion mixture into the cooked scrambled egg and serve.

Mushroom Lover's Omelet

Ingredients

Cooking spray

1 cup chopped fresh mushrooms – Preferably a combo of 2 or more different types like button and Portobello's.

1 cup liquid egg substitute

1 finely chopped onion

¼ tsp thyme

¼ tsp basil

1 tbsp parsley

Salt and freshly ground pepper to taste

Preparation

- In a medium sized skillet sauté onions and mushrooms for about 3 min. remove from heat.
- Add the basil, parsley, thyme, salt and pepper and then remove sautéed mix from skillet.
- Spray the skillet with more cooking spray and pour in 1/2 of the egg substitute. Cook until lightly browned on the bottom and then flip over to cook the opposite side.
- Once cooked, place 1/2 of the sautéed mix onto the omelet and fold in half.

- Remove omelet from skillet and store in oven or just cover.
- Use the rest of the egg and sautéed mix to make the second omelet.

Breakfast Burrito

Ingredients

2 tbsp diced onions

½ tbsp canned chopped green chilies

½ cup egg substitute

1 tbsp Monterey Jack cheese (fat free)

Salt and ground black pepper to taste

A few drops of hot pepper sauce (to taste)

1x 98% fat-free flour tortilla (heated)

Preparation

- After spraying cooking spray onto a skillet, sauté onions and chilies.
- Combine egg substitute, cheese, pepper, and pepper sauce and whisk.
- Pour the mixture into the skillet and cook for approximately 4 minutes.
- Place the egg mixture along the middle of the tortilla. Fold up the bottom part and then roll the sides over. Breakfast is served!

Strawberry Pancakes

Ingredients

4 egg whites

1/2 cup rolled oats

3 tsp strawberry jam – sugar free

1 tbsp grapeseed oil

Cooking spray

Preparation

- Place egg whites, strawberry jam, oil and oats in a blender and mix until smooth.
- Coat skillet with cooking spray and heat. Once heated pour 1/2 of the prepared batter to make your first pancake. Cook each side for about 2 min until golden brown.
- Repeat process to make second pancake.

Smoked Salmon and Vegetable Omelet

Ingredients

4 medium sized eggs

1/4 cup smoked salmon, chopped

1 chopped tomatoes

1/2 chopped onion

1/4 cup finely chopped spinach

1/2 cup chopped mushrooms

1 slice rye break

Preparation

- In a skillet heat oil and sauté' onions, mushrooms, spinach, and tomatoes. Remove from heat.
- Beat eggs in a separate bowl and then add smoked salmon pieces. Pour mixture over sautéed vegetables and cook until omelet is golden brown.
- Serve with rye break.

Banana Muffins With Nutmeg Surprise

Ingredients

6 mashed and peeled ripe bananas

3 cups whole wheat self-rising flour

1 1/2 tsp baking soda

1/2 cup butter

8 tbsp water

1 1/2 cups artificial sweetener

1 cup egg substitute

1 tsp salt

1 tbsp ground nutmeg

1 tsp vanilla extract

Preparation

- Preheat oven to 374 deg. F (190 deg. Celsius) and grease a muffin pan big enough to make about 20 muffins.
- Place the flour, baking soda, butter, water, sweetener, egg substitute, vanilla, nutmeg and salt in large bowl and combine. Once combined fold in mashed banana.
- Take your batter and fill each muffin cup to the 3/4 mark.

- Place in preheated oven and bake for about 15 minutes – or less if you don't want the banana to be cooked too much.

Black Bean and Salsa Omelet

Ingredients

2 whole eggs and 4 egg whites

1/3 cup reduced fat cheddar cheese

1/4 cup salsa

1 medium sized chopped tomato

1 cup canned black beans drained

1/4 chopped avocado pear

Salt and ground black pepper to taste

Cooking spray

Preparation

- Place whole eggs and egg whites in a bowl and whisk together. Add desired amount of salt and pepper.
- Spray cooking spray on your pan and heat over medium heat. Pour the egg mixture into heated pan and cook for around 3 min until almost done.
- At this point sprinkle the salsa, cheese, black beans and 1/2 of the chopped tomato over the egg and continue to cook for an additional 3 min. It is ready when the egg is cooked through and the cheese is nicely melted.

- Fold your cooked omelet in half and remove from the pan. Once plated top with avocado pieces and remaining tomato.

Lunch Recipes

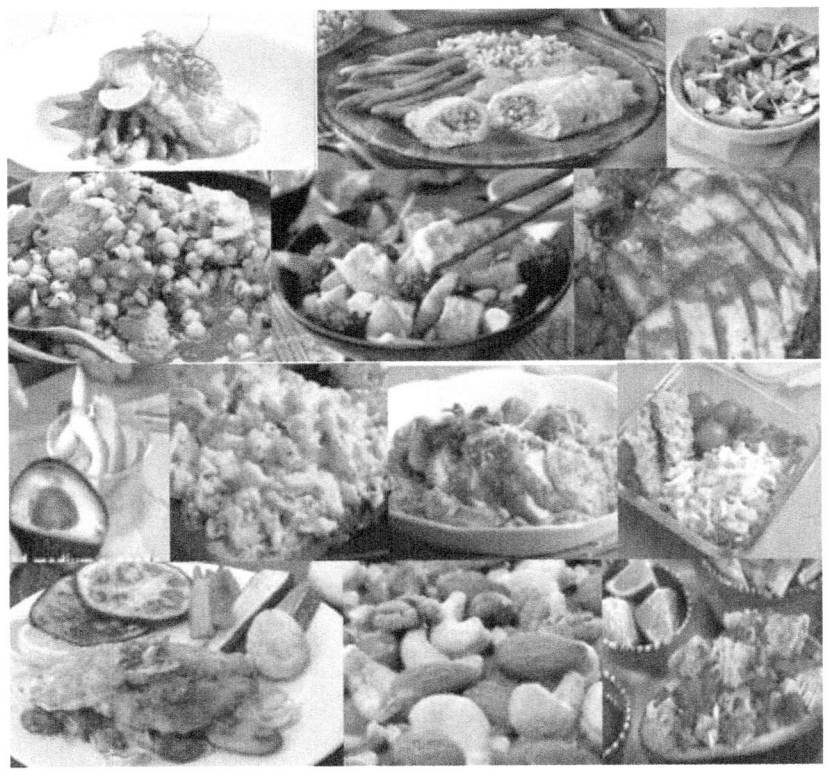

Delicious Chicken Tortilla

Ingredients

1 sliced chicken breast

1 tsp olive oil

1 finely chopped onion

1roughly chopped red or green pepper

A few small tortillas

1 peeled and grated carrot

1 cup of lettuce

14 oz. drained kidney beans

1 tbsp crème fraiche

Salt and pepper

Preparation

- Fry the onion and pepper in the tsp of olive oil for approximately 2 minutes.
- Add the chicken pieces and continue frying until the chicken is cooked and nicely browned.
- In a separate bowl combine and crème fraiche and kidney beans and mash.

- Spread the mixture onto a few tortillas and then add the chicken, lettuce leaves and carrots before you roll it up. Guaranteed to be delicious!

American Style Waldorf Salad

Ingredients

1 cup red seedless grapes (cut in half)

2 tbsp lemon juice

½ cup low fat mayonnaise

2 finely chopped sticks of celery

4 apples cut into chunky pieces

2 tbsp chopped walnuts

Preparation

- Place the grapes, celery, apples and walnuts into a salad bowl.
- In a separate bowl combine the mayonnaise and lemon juice.
- Drizzle your dressing over the salad and toss.

Thai Chicken Noodle Salad

Ingredients

2 chopped chicken breasts

2 chopped cloves of garlic

1 lime (use juice and zest)

1 tsp oil

2 tbsp chopped coriander

1 orange (use juice and zest)

¼ cucumber sliced

½ chopped red chili

3 oz. halved blanched beans

1 cup cooked noodles

3 sliced spring onions

I tsp honey

Preparation

- Place the chicken in a medium sized dish and cover with the juice and zest from the lime. Place in the refrigerator and leave to marinate for approximately 30 min.

- Place the tsp of olive oil in a frying pan and fry the garlic and chicken until the chicken is properly cooked (should take about 8 min).
- In a large bowl combine the onion, coriander, beans, cucumber, noodles and chili.
- Make a dressing out of the honey and orange and drizzle over salad
- To serve, place salad in plates and finish off by placing the fried chicken on top.

Turkey Burger Drizzled With Mango Chutney

Ingredients

1 long whole wheat baguette

1 sliced large red onion

¼ tsp salt

1 lb ground turkey that is 93% lean

4 tbsp mango chutney

Preparation

- Preheat your grill to medium high
- Cut your long whole wheat baguette into four equal pieces. Slice the pieces in half and then remove about half of the soft bread from the inside.
- In a medium sized bowl combine the onions, turkey, salt, and 1 tbsp. chutney and mix thoroughly until properly combined. Form 4 turkey burgers out of the mixture. They should be about ½ inch thick.
- Place the burgers onto the hot grill and grill each side for approximately 3 to 4 minutes.
- Once done remove the burgers and place the remaining onion slices on the grill. Grill them for a few minutes until they have browned a little.

- Place the grilled burgers and onions onto your baguettes and drizzle with the remaining mango chutney.

Club Salad

Ingredients

1 cup of fat-free salad dressing

2 tbsp chopped onions

2 tbsp shredded chives

¼ tsp salt

½ tsp dry mustard

¼ shredded parsley

¼ cup tarragon vinegar

Pinch of ground black pepper

2 cups chopped lettuce leaves

2 cooked chicken breasts, cubes

2 tomatoes

5 slices of grilled bacon (remove fat before grilling)

Preparation

- In a medium sized bowl combine the dressing, vinegar, parsley, onions, chives, mustard, salt and pepper. Place in the refrigerator and allow to infuse for a few hours.

- Place greens in a salad bowl and cubed chicken pieces right in the center. Coat the greens and chicken with your dressing and finish off by evenly distributing the slices of tomato and bacon bits.

Sweet And Sour Chicken Salad

Ingredients

4 large chicken breasts (boneless and skinless)

Teriyaki sauce (enough to marinate chicken in)

8 won tons

1 head lettuce chopped

2 tbsp + 2 tsp vinegar

3 tbsp + 2 tsp canola oil

¾ tsp paprika

Ground black pepper

1 tbsp sweet and sour sauce

1 tbsp sesame seeds (toasted)

1 tsp salt

¼ cup green onions

Preparation

- Marinate chicken pieces in Teriyaki sauce for a few hours before baking or placing in microwave until cooked through. Cut into cubes.
- Fry won ton in 1 tbsp canola oil and drain.

- Combine the vinegar, remaining canola oil, paprika, black pepper, sweet and sour sauce and salt in a pot and bring to a boil. Once boiling starts turn off heat and allow to cool.
- In a salad bowl combine the lettuce, chicken, sesame seeds, and green onions.
- Just before serving add the dressing and won tons and your sticky delicious salad is ready!

Whole Wheat Crab Sandwich

Ingredients

2 whole wheat rolls

2 tsp butter

1 clove chopped garlic

1 egg

Cayenne pepper to taste

1 tbsp milk

Pinch of salt

1 tbsp canola oil

1 cup crab meat, flaked (alternatively you can use shrimp or lobster)

Tabasco sauce to taste (optional)

Preparation

- Cut whole wheat rolls in half and butter on all sides.
- In a saucepan sauté the garlic in canola oil until it starts to brown. Now add the crab meat and continue to cook over low heat, stirring from time to time.
- In a separate bowl combine the egg (must be beaten), cayenne, Tabasco, milk, and salt.

- Slowly add this mixture to the crab meat and keep stirring until the crab starts holding together.
- Divide your crab meat into two portions and place on whole wheat rolls just before serving.

Hot Noodle Salad On A Bed Of Cold Lettuce

Ingredients

1 cup whole grain noodles

3 cups fresh asparagus (cut in 1 inch. Pieces)

3 roughly chopped tomatoes

1 cup roughly chopped green bell pepper

½ cup beef broth (canned)

2 tbsp canola oil

1 large clove of garlic (pressed)

1 head of lettuce

Salt and pepper to taste

Handful of parmesan cheese

Preparation

- Cook noodles according to package instruction.
- Add asparagus and bell peppers two minutes before the noodles are done.
- In a salad bowl place chopped lettuce and tomatoes and sprinkle with salt and pepper.
- Place the oil, garlic and broth in a microwaveable bowl and heat.

- Once noodles and vegetables are done, drain and place on top of lettuce. Finish off by pouring hot oil dressing over.
- Sprinkle parmesan cheese on the top.

Whole Wheat Roll Topped With Avo And Shrimp

Ingredients

2 large avocados

1 cup low-fat softened cream cheese

2 tbsp low fat mayonnaise

¼ tsp salt

1 tbsp chopped green onions

6 whole wheat rolls

18 shrimps or scallops

¼ tsp dill weed

2 tbsp prepared mustard

Preparation

- Remove skin and seeds from avocados and slice into large rings.
- Place the cream cheese, mayonnaise, salt, mustard, dill week, green onions and mustard in a bowl and mix using an electric mixer (alternatively use a blender).
- Cut your whole wheat rolls in half and liberally spread the cream cheese mixture on all sides.
- Fill the rolls with shrimp and avocado rings and finish off by sprinkling some dill over the top. Serves 6.

Corn, Avo And Brown Rice Salad

Ingredients

3 cups cooked brown rice

½ cup toasted almonds

1 avocado

2 ears of cooked corn

1 tsp lemon juice

1 tsp canola oil

1 tsp brown rice vinegar

1 tsp tamari soy sauce

4 chopped large lettuce leaves

Preparation

- Cook rice according to package instructions
- Peel the avo and pit before mashing with the cooked rice.
- Remove the corn from the cob and add to the mixture. Also add the onions and almonds.
- In a small bowl combine the oil, vinegar, lemon juice, and tamari sauce. Mix together and pour all over salad. Serve chilled.

Chicken And Berry Salad

Ingredients

1 cup chicken strips

1 cup blueberries

1 cup finely grated carrots

1 medium sized bag crisp lettuce

1 tsp canola oil

1 tsp cayenne pepper

1/2 tsp ginger

1/2 cup raspberries

Preparation

- Combine the cayenne pepper and ginger and spice chicken strips before cooking in a pan for approximately 5 minutes.
- In a large salad bowl combine the lettuce, carrots, blueberries, raspberries and cooked chicken strips. Drizzle with any fat free dressing and add salt and pepper to taste.

Turkey And Coleslaw Sandwich

Ingredients

2 cups grated carrot and cabbage (mixed)

2 tbsp low fat Italian salad dressing

2 slices of rye bread

9 oz. thinly slices turkey breast (cooked)

3 slices provolone cheese

1 thinly sliced tomato

Cucumber slices

Preparation

- Place coleslaw mix in a bowl and combine with Italian dressing.
- Place rye bread slices on a plate and top with turkey, cheese slices, tomato, coleslaw, and cucumber slices.
- Close sandwich and toast in a heated pan – 4 min per side or until cheese is melted.

Thai Vegetable Pizza

Ingredients

1 Italian bread shell (18 inch)\

1/2 cup chopped button mushrooms (or shitake)

2 tbsp chopped green 1/3 cup fresh pea pods cut into thin strips

2 tbsp grated carrot

2 tbsp chopped green onion

Non stick cooking spray

3 tbsp peanut sauce

1 tbsp roughly diced peanuts

A few cilantro leaves

Preparation

- Preheat oven to 446 deg. F (230 deg. Celsius) and place Italian bread shell on a baking sheet and bake for a few minutes until crisp.
- Coat a skillet with the nonstick cooking spray and add pea pods, mushroom, onions and carrot. Cook for 4 minutes.
- Drizzle peanut sauce over crispy Italian bread shell and spread evenly. Top with cooked vegetable mix. To finish off sprinkle with peanuts and add Cilantro leaves.

Chicken, Red Pepper And Avocado Focaccia

Ingredients

18 inch focaccia

1/2 cup roasted red sweet peppers, sliced

4 thick slices roast chicken (cooked)

1/3 cup light mayonnaise

1/3 cup mashed avocado

Preparation

- Cut focaccia in half and spread both sides with low fat mayonnaise.
- Top with roast chicken slices, red peppers and mashed avocado. Simple yet delicious.

Thai Style Pancakes

Ingredients

Pancakes

1/2 cup flour

1 tsp Canola Oil

1 1/4 cup skim milk

1 beaten egg

Filling

350 g chicken breast (boneless and skinless) strips

1/4 cup cashew nuts (broken in half)

2 tsp canola oil

1 crushed garlic clove

1 tsp chopped fresh ginger

2 thinly sliced celery sticks

2 carrots, sliced into long thin pieces

1 cup chopped cabbage

1/2 tsp sesame oil

1 tbsp soy sauce

Zest from one medium sized orange

Preparation

- To make pancakes combine the egg and milk and place to one side. Sift the flour into a bowl and then add the egg mixture and whisk until combined. Add salt and pepper to taste. Batter should be smooth but not too runny.

- Heat a little oil in a pan and then spoon some of the batter into the heated pan to make your pancake. Cook the first side for about 2 min, or until you start seeing bubbles from. Flip the pancake and cook the other side for about a minute until golden brown. Repeat the process until all pancakes are done – the batter is enough for eight pancakes.

- To make the filling, start by heating a wok. Add cashew nuts and stir fry for a few minutes. Remove and set aside.

- Heat a little oil in the same wok and then add chicken, ginger and garlic. Fry for at least 4 minutes before adding the celery, carrots, and cabbage. Slowly add the soy sauce, sesame oil and zest. Fry for an extra 4 minutes and then add crunchy cashew nuts.

- Spoon some of the stir fry mixture into each of the 8 pancakes and roll to close. Serve with extra soy sauce.

Vegetarian Open Sandwich

Ingredients

2 tsp Dijon mustard

1/4 cup grated carrot

1/2 cup broccoli florets (small)

2 toasted whole-wheat English Muffins

1/4 cup roughly chopped red bell pepper

1/2 cup shredded Monterey Jack Cheese (Low Fat)

Preparation

- Turn on oven (grill)
- Spread Dijon mustard over all sides of English Muffin and top with broccoli, carrots and bell peppers. Finish of with shredded cheese.
- Place under grill for a few min, or until cheese has melted.

Dinner Recipes

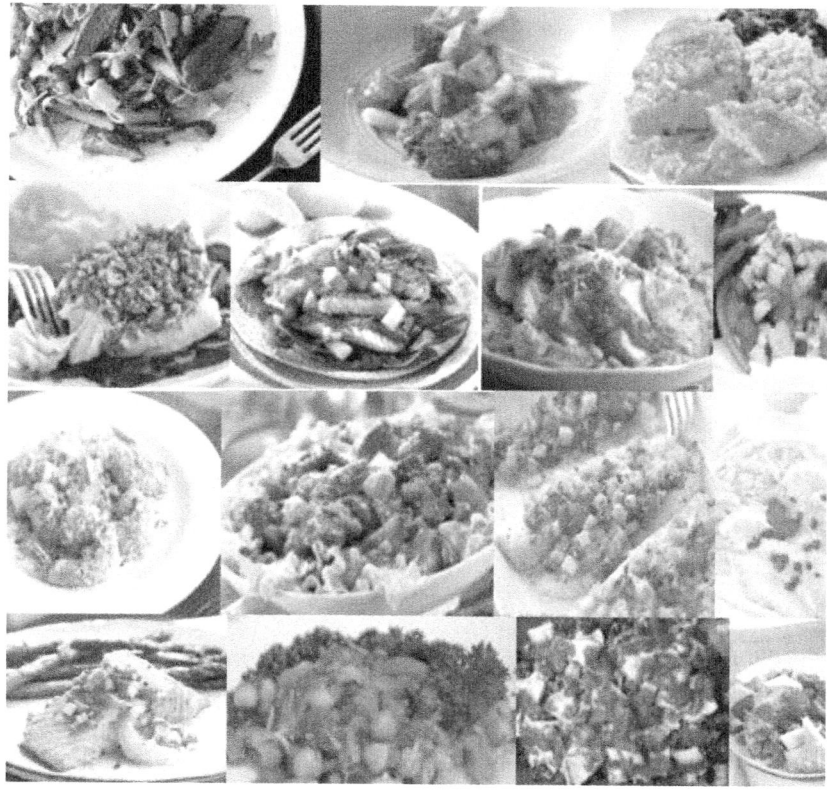

Hearty Sweet Potato Soup With Red Pepper

Ingredients

1 lb peeled cubed sweet potato

2 seeded and cubed red peppers

2 chopped cloves of garlic

1 chopped onion

10 ounces (300ml) dry white wine

41 ounces (1.2 L) chicken or vegetable stock (Light)

Salt and Pepper to taste

Bread to serve with soup

Preparation

- Put the peeled cubed sweet potato, red peppers, garlic, onion, chicken/vegetable stock and wine into a saucepan and bring to the boil.
- Allow to simmer for 30 min or until the vegetables are soft.
- Pour the mixture into a food processor or blender and blend until smooth and creamy. Serve warm with bread.

Spinach And Green Pea Soup

Ingredients

1 cup finely sliced fresh spinach

1 chopped stick of celery

1.5 ounces finely chopped cabbage

½ finely shredded lettuce

2 1/2 cups frozen or fresh peas (podded)

2 crushed cloves of garlic

1 finely chopped leek

2 tbsp olive oil

1 tbsp finely chopped parsley

2/3 ounce (20 ml) shredded fresh mint

Salt and pepper to taste

41 ounces (1.2 L) chicken stock

2 slices of rindless back bacon

½ carton mustard and cress

Preparation

- Place the leek, garlic, peas, bacon and stock in a large saucepan and bring to the boil. Allow to simmer for 20 min.
- When the first mixture is almost ready heat oil in a frying pan and add the lettuce, spinach, cabbage, herbs and celery. Cover and sweat over low heat until tender.
- Now transfer the pea mixture into a blender and process until smooth.
- Combine the blended mixture with the vegetables and herbs.
- Season with salt and pepper and serve with bread.

Spaghetti With Creamy Smoked Salmon

Ingredients

1 cup finely chopped mushrooms

8 fl oz dry white wine

2 tbsp olive oil

8 oz thinly sliced smoked salmon

10 fl oz. low fat soya cream (unsweetened)

1 ½ tsp fresh dill

1 tbsp fresh chives

Lemon Juice

10 oz (about 2 cups) spaghetti

Sea salt and Black pepper for seasoning

Preparation

- In a large saucepan heat the oil and then lightly fry the mushrooms.
- Add the white wine and bring to a boil. Boil for 5 min. or until the wine has reduced a lot.
- Stir the soya cream and herbs into the mixture and then add the salmon and reheat. (Be sure not to boil)
- Add some lemon juice and black pepper to taste and cover.

- Cook the spaghetti in a pot of salted boiling water until ready.
- Drain the spaghetti and finish off by combining with the salmon sauce.
- Garnish with chives.

Chicken And Vegetable Dish - Two Meals In One!

Ingredients

5 lb chicken

2 chopped celery sticks

3 thickly sliced carrots

2 onions cut in 4 pieces

1 turnip cut into thick slices

½ cup mushrooms

Handful of fresh parsley

4 bay leaves

1 tsp dried thyme

1 cup pasta (wholemeal)

Salt and black pepper

Whole wheat bread

Preparation

- Start by cutting all excess fat off the chicken and then place it in a casserole dish with all the herbs and vegetables.

- Add enough water to cover and bring to the boil. Once the water has started boiling, lower the temperature and simmer for approximately 2.5 hours.
- Once cooked carefully carve the chicken and be sure to get rid of the skin and bones. Small remaining pieces of chicken can be placed back into the pan.
- Serve the tender chicken with some of the cooked vegetables.
- The remaining broth in the pan can be stored and left to chill for use the next day. Before storing it remove any large pieces of thyme and parsley.
- When you are ready to prepare your next dish remove the broth from the refrigerator and first remove the fat that would have solidified on the top.
- Reheat the soup. Once it starts boiling add the pasta.
- Season with salt and pepper and serve with a few slices of whole wheat bread.

Hearty Winter Chicken Stew

Ingredients

4 chicken thighs – cut in half and skinned

2 tsp oil

12 new potatoes cut in half

1 small chopped up cabbage

1 quartered onion

1 tbsp flour with added salt and pepper

1 crushed clove of garlic

1 peeled and chopped carrot

10 fl oz. chicken stock

1 tsp Black Pepper

Preparation

- Rub the flour all over the chicken thighs before placing in a pan with oil and browning. Once browned remove from the pan and set aside.
- In the same pan fry the garlic and all the vegetables except the cabbage for 5 minutes.
- Add the chicken stock.

- Take the chicken that you set aside and add to the vegetable and stock mixture.
- Bring the stew to a boil. Once it has started boiling turn down the heat and allow to simmer f or 30 minutes.
- Finally, add the cabbage and the pepper and allow to cook for 5 more minutes before serving.

Chicken And Broccoli Pasta

Ingredients

2 ½ cups of whole grain pasta

3 cups broccoli

4 skinless chicken breast halves cut into small pieces

1 minced clove garlic

1 ¼ cup light mayonnaise

¼ tsp ground black pepper

2 tbsp olive oil

2 tbsp shredded parmesan cheese

1 tsp adobo seasoning

Preparation

- Cook pasta according to package instruction and in the last five minutes add the broccoli. Now drain the pasta and broccoli and put it back into the pot (preferably a Dutch oven)
- Place the chicken pieces in a separate bowl and coat with the adobo seasoning.
- Heat your olive oil in a skillet and fry the garlic for around 30 sec. Now add the coated chicken pieces and cook until they are golden brown. This should take between 3 and 4 minutes.

- Once the chicken is cooked add it to the pasta and broccoli in the Dutch oven. Mix in the pepper and mayonnaise and continue cooking over low heat until, stirring from time to time.
- Before serving sprinkle Parmesan Cheese over the dish.

Creamy Vegetable And Shrimp Pasta

Ingredients

1 1/2 cups whole wheat pasta

12 oz raw shrimp – devein, peel and cut into 1 inch pieces

3 cloves of roughly chopped garlic

1 cup peas

1 bunch sliced asparagus

1 thinly sliced red pepper

1 ½ cups low fat or non-fat yoghurt

1 ¼ tsp kosher salt

3 tbsp lemon juice

½ tsp ground black pepper

¼ toasted pine nuts

¼ cup chopped parsley

1 tbsp olive oil

Preparation

• Bring a medium sized pot of water to the boil and then add the spaghetti. Cook according to package instructions.

- Once the spaghetti is 2 minutes from being done add the bell pepper, peas, shrimp and asparagus and cook until shrimp is done and then drain.
- In a separate bowl combine and mash the salt and garlic to form a paste.
- Stir the yoghurt, lemon juice, oil, parsley and pepper into the paste.
- Toss everything together – the pasta mixture with the paste - and sprinkle with nuts if you like.

Crunchy Dijon Flavored Chicken Breasts Covered In Mushrooms

Ingredients

4 skinless boneless chicken breasts

2 tbsp olive oil

½ tsp salt

¼ tsp pepper

¼ cup all-purpose flour

1 tin of sliced mushrooms

½ cup roasted garlic seasoned chicken broth

1 ½ tbsp. Dijon mustard

Preparation

- Place chicken pieces between a sheet of plastic wrap and then using a rolling pin or meat pin, pound the meat until it is ¼ inch thick.
- Combine the salt, pepper, and flour in a shallow dish.
- Dip the chicken breasts in the flour mixture – make sure they are properly coated.
- In a medium sized pan heat the olive oil and proceed to fry the chicken pieces for about 6 to 8 minutes. You only need to turn the chicken once.

- Remove the chicken pieces and pour the broth into the pan. Once the broth has started boiling stir in the mushrooms and mustard and allow to cook until the broth has thickened somewhat.
- Finish off by pouring the delicious broth over the crispy chicken pieces. This dish is guaranteed to be a hit every time!

Butternut Soup

Ingredients

1 large butternut squash

2 tbsp butter (unsalted)

1 chopped onion

Nutmeg to taste

6 cups chicken stock

Salt

Freshly ground black pepper

Preparation

- Peel and seed the butternut and then cut into chunks.
- Melt the butter in a large pot and fry the onions for a few minutes until they start to brown.
- Add your chunks of butternut and the chicken stock and bring to a simmer.
- Allow to simmer between 15 and 20 minutes or until the butternut is cooked through. It needs to be tender.
- Remove the chunky pieces of squash and place them in a blender to make a puree.
- Once blended place the squash back into the pot and finish off by seasoning with salt, pepper and nutmeg.

Creamy Tomato Soup With A Peanut Surprise

Ingredients

1 tbsp olive oil

1 chopped onion

1 finely chopped green bell pepper

1 can crushed tomatoes

4 cups low-sodium chicken broth

¼ tsp Stevia powdered extract (2-3 drops Stevia liquid concentrate)

1 finely chopped celery stalk

1 chopped clove of garlic

1/2 tsp curry powder

1/2 tsp paprika

1/8 tsp cayenne pepper

Salt and black ground pepper to taste

1/3 cup peanut butter (preferably smooth)

Preparation

- Heat the olive oil in a medium sized pan and fry the onions, peppers and celery for about 5 minutes. Now add the paprika, curry powder, garlic, 1 tsp salt and cayenne pepper and cook for a further 2 minutes.

- Now add the chicken broth, Stevia, crushed tomatoes, and 1 cup of water. Using a whisk slowly add the peanut butter until properly blended.
- Once the soup starts to boil, turn down the heat and simmer for a further 30 minutes stirring every now and then. The soup should have thickened by the time its ready.
- Pour the soup into a blender and blend until a puree forms. Add salt and pepper to taste.

Pork Tenderloin

Ingredients

2 pork tenderloins

2 tbsp chili powder

¼ tsp of ground ginger, thyme and pepper (1/4 tsp of each)

1 tsp salt

Preparation

- In a small bowl combine all the spices.
- Run the spices all over the tenderloin to season. Cover and place in the fridge for a few hours.
- Grill tenderloins over medium heat for 30 to 40 minutes until cooked through.

Pork Chops Basted In A Sweet Orange Sauce

Ingredients

6 thick pork loin chops

1 tbsp vegetable oil

1 Tbsp Stevia powdered extract (1 tsp Stevia liquid concentrate)

¾ cup water

½ tsp pepper

½ tsp paprika

1 ¼ tsp salt

1 orange (zest and then peel and cut into pieces)

1 cup orange juice (fresh)

1 tbsp cornstarch

12 cloves

½ tsp cinnamon

Preparation

- In a large pan heat oil and then brown pork on both sides. Now add the water, salt, paprika, and pepper and bring to a boil. Turn down the heat and allow to cook for 40 minutes. Turn the chops at least once during this time.

- In a separate saucepan add orange juice, 1 tbsp orange zest , Steviastarch, cloves, cinnamon and leftover salt. Allow to cook until thick and then add orange pieces.
- Pour this delicious sauce over your pork chops and serve with vegetables of your choice.

Grilled Chicken Breasts – Mediterranean Style

Ingredients

4 large chicken breasts

1 tsp oregano leaves

2 tbsp grated lemon peel

1 chopped red onion

20 kalamata olives (pitted)

4 Roma tomatoes (plum) quartered

1/2 cup low fat feta cheese (preferably tomato and basil flavored)

Preparation

- Cut 4 large pieces of heavy duty foil that you will be using for grilling the chicken (18 by 12 inch). Preheat Grill.
- Lay out the sheets of foil and on each one place a chicken breast, slices of tomato, a tbsp of chopped onion, and 5 olives. Once that is done top each chicken breast with ¼ cup of the feta cheese.
- Now wrap up each chicken breast in the foil by pulling the sides over. Seal on all sides in preparation for grilling.
- Place the packages on the grill over medium heat and allow to cool for approximately 25 minutes, turning halfway through the

cooking time (after about 12 minutes). Guaranteed to be tender and delicious!

Pork Roast With Berry Glaze

Ingredients

1 large pork loin

2 cups raspberries

2 cups blackberries

1 tsp thyme

2 tbsp of crushed pecans

Preparation

- Place blackberries and raspberries in a blender and blend until liquid consistency has formed.
- Preheat your oven to 392 deg. F (200 deg. Celsius).
- Place pork in oven pan and Rub thyme all over before topping with liquidized berries.
- Cover foil and bake for approximately 4 hours or until loin is tender.
- Serve with your favorite vegetables.

Cabbage Rolls Stuffed With Pork And Veggies

Ingredients

7 oz. lean minced pork

2 cups cooked brown rice

8 big cabbage leaves

1 tsp olive oil

1 large carrot, grated

1 chopped brown onion

1 finely diced celery stalk

1 tbsp tomato paste

2 tsp ground cumin

1 tsp ground coriander

1/2 tsp ground allspice

2 crushed garlic cloves

1/3 cup baby rocket leaves

Tomato Sauce

1 1/2 cups canned crushed tomatoes

1/2 cup chicken stock (reduced salt)

2 crushed cloves garlic

1 tbsp shredded fresh flat-leaf parsley

Preparation

- Cook cabbage leaves by either steaming or boiling. Once cooked, rinse and drain and place on absorbent paper to get rid of excess moisture.
- In a large saucepan fry onions, carrots, celery and garlic for about 5 min. Now add paste and pork and keep frying until pork has browned.
- Once the pork has browned add the remaining spices and stir to combine.
- Slowly stir in rice. Now remove from heat and allow to cool for a few minutes.
- Distribute the rice mixture amongst the cabbage leaves and carefully roll each one making sure to fold in all edges.
- Cook the rolls for 10 minutes over either a bamboo steamer lined with baking paper or over a large pot of simmering water. Each roll must be cooked and heated all the way through.
- To make tomato sauce, place undrained tomatoes, garlic and stock in a small pan. Once the mixture starts to boil, reduce heat and simmer uncovered for about 10 minutes. Once done stir in parsley.

Spicy Lamb Served With Barley Salad

Ingredients

1 tbsp crushed coriander seeds

1/2 tsp dried chili flakes

2 cloves crushed garlic

1 lb lamb backstraps

1 cup pearl barley

1/4 teaspoon ground turmeric

1/3 cup each loosely packed fresh mint and coriander leaves

1 chopped small red onion

1 cup cherry tomatoes – cut in half

1/4 cup lemon juice

2 tsp olive oil

Preparation

- Make the lamb spice by combining the chili, garlic and seeds. Once combined rub spice all over lamb. Place in the refrigerator for 30 min.
- Place barley in large pot and boil for approximately 20 min. Rinse and drain once cooked.

- Cook lamb on a grill to your liking. Once done put to one side and allow to stand for few minutes before slicing into thick pieces.
- Place the rest of the ingredients in a large bowl and add cooked barley.
- Serve tender pieces of lamb with barley salad.

Creamy Marinara Pasta

Ingredients

1 cup linguine pasta

14 oz. marinara mix

1 small finely diced brown onion

2 garlic cloves, crushed

1 fresh small chopped red thai chilli

1 can diced tomatoes

1/4 cup water

1/3 cup coarsely chopped fresh flat-leaf parsley

Preparation

- Cook pasta according to package instructions.
- While the pasta is cooking, heat some oil in a large saucepan and cook marinara for about 2 minutes. Remove and place in separate dish.
- Using the same pan fry the onions, chili and garlic for 5 minutes. Now add the can of tomatoes and the water and continue cooking for an additional 5 minutes.
- Transfer marinara back to pan and carry on cooking for 2 minutes, stirring occasionally. Finish off by adding parsley.
- Plate pasta and top with delicious marinara mix.

Spicy Kebabs With Fluffy Couscous

Ingredients

1/2 cup diced fresh coriander

1 lb fish fillets (firm, white, and skinless) – cut into 3cm pieces

1 cup chicken stock (reduced salt)

2 cloves garlic, crushed

1 tbsp olive oil

2 small red Thai chilies, chopped

1/4 cup lemon juice

1/2 cup water

1 1/2 cups couscous

1/2 cup fresh coriander

1 tbsp preserved lemon, finely chopped

1/4 cup slivered almonds, toasted

Preparation

- Place the oil, garlic, coriander, chili and lemon juice in a large bowl. Add fish pieces and coat with spice mix.

- Using 8 skewers make kebabs out of the fish fillets (should make about 8) and place on a try. Cover and place in fridge for 40 minutes.
- Heat an oiled grill plate (or barbeque) and allow kebabs to cook for about 5 minutes.
- Pour stock and the water into a pot and bring to the boil. Remove from heat and add couscous. Cover and allow to stand for 5 minutes, or until the liquid is absorbed. After 5 minutes, fluff the couscous using a fork. Finish off by adding what was left of the coriander spice mix, coriander leaves, lemon and nuts to the couscous. Serve couscous with grilled fish kebabs.

Thai Chicken Stir Fry

Ingredients

14 oz. sliced chicken breast fillets

11/2 cups doongara rice

3 cups water

1 tsp sesame oil

1/4 cup soy sauce (reduced salt)

1/4 cup lime juice

1 cup fresh baby corn

1/4 cup water (extra)

2 tbsp honey

2 chopped red Thai chilies

2 tsp corn flour

2 tsp lime rind, finely grated

3 cups bean sprouts

2 cups fresh Thai basil leaves

1 cup fresh coriander

1 tbsp peanut oil

3 cloves garlic, crushed

2 finely sliced red onions

Preparation

- To make a marinade, combine honey, chili, sesame oil, cornflour, juice and sauce in bowl. Place chicken in mixture and coat completely. Cover and place in fridge for at least an hour.
- Cook rice according to package instructions.
- Remove chicken from marinade. Keep marinade
- Brown the chicken in a wok, in batches using 1/2 of the peanut oil. Remove from wok and place to one side. Using the rest of the peanut oil fry the onion, garlic, corn and tender, but not overcooked. Place browned chicken back into the wok with the leftover marinade, extra water and rind. Keep frying until the chicken is cooked through.
- Before serving sprinkle with herbs and sprouts. Serve delicious chicken and veggie mix with rice.

Dessert Recipes

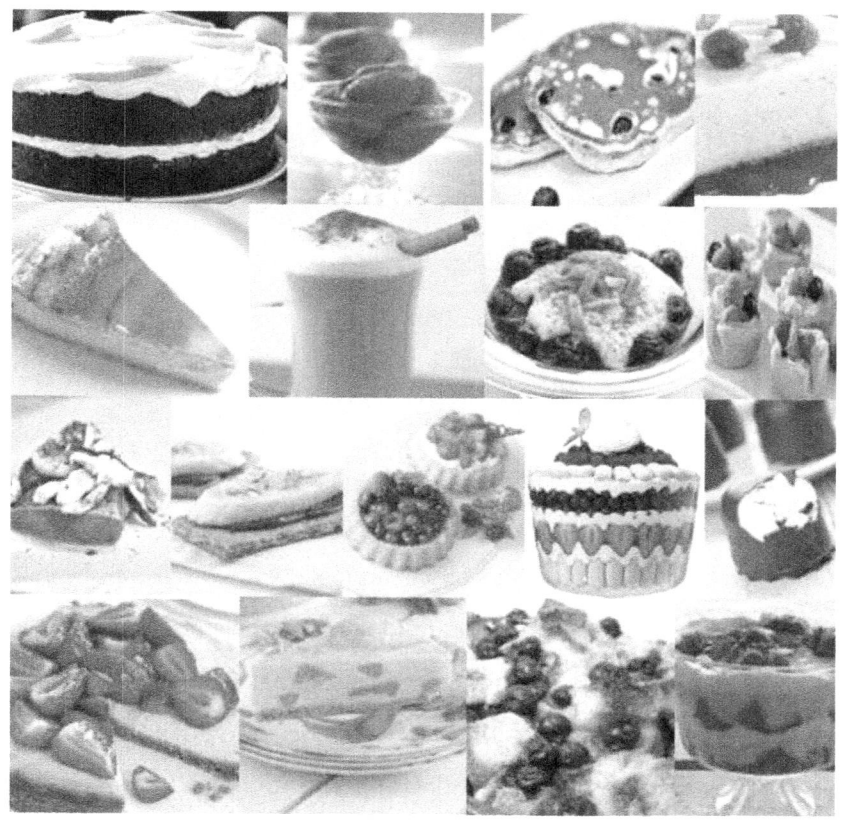

Cranberry Rice Pudding

Ingredients

1 ¼ cups rice milk

1/3 cup short grain rice

¼ cup cranberries

1 vanilla pod

Preparation

- Preheat your over to 302 deg. F (150 deg. Celsius)
- Pour the rice milk into a medium sized saucepan as well as the vanilla pod. When the milk has almost reached boiling point remove it from the stove and allow the milk and vanilla to combine for 10 minutes. Remove the vanilla pod.
- Place the rice and cranberries into a baking dish and proceed to pour the milk into the dish. Mix and then bake in the oven for about 2 ½ to 3 hours. Stir from time to time. This dessert can be served either warm or cold.

Orange Chocolate Mousse

Ingredients

1 cup dark chocolate squares

Rind and juice from 1 ½ large oranges

4 separated eggs

1 tsp gelatine (powder)

4 tbsp brandy

6 tbsp soya cream

Preparation

- Heat water in a pan over the stove and then place a heatproof bowl over the pan to melt the chocolate.
- In a separate heatproof brown add 2 tbsp of orange juice and sprinkle the gelatin powder on top.
- Once the gelatin has reached a spongy consistency stir until it has completely dissolved.
- Allow the chocolate to cook over the pan of hot water before you mix in the egg yolks, orange rind, brandy, soya cream and rind. Stir in the gelatin and the remaining orange juice and place to one side.
- In a medium sized bowl whisk the egg whites until they are fluffy and then proceed to fold them into the chocolate and orange mixture.

- Pour the mixture into the bowls or glasses you plan on serving them in. Place into the refrigerator until chilled.

Creamy Strawberry Pita

Ingredients

1 cup chopped strawberries

3 tbsp of low fat cream cheese

1 whole wheat pita bread

Preparation

- In a bowl combine the ¼ cup of strawberries with cream cheese. Mix together and mash the berries in the process.
- Cut open the pita and spread half of the strawberry mixture inside and on both sides of the pita. Use the remaining strawberries to fill the pita.
- Spray pita with non-stick spray and grill in pan on both sides until golden brown.
- Heat a cast iron pan or skillet to warm. Spray sandwich with non-stick spray and grill both sides until golden. Serve warm. So simple yet so delicious!

Delicious Diabetic Tiramisu

Ingredients

1 tablespoon instant coffee powder

3/4 cup boiling water

1 cup low-fat ricotta cheese

1 ½ Stevia powdered extract (12-18 drops Stevia liquid concentrate)

1/2 cup light sour cream

2 tbsp Marsala

9 halved sponge-fingers

2 tsp cocoa powder

Preparation

- Dissolve coffee in boiling water and stir in Marsala.
- Divide the biscuit halves between three 6 ounce (180ml) glasses (3 each) and then drizzle the coffee over them
- Place the stevia, sour cream and cheese in medium sized bowl and combine with electric mixer. You can stop once it starts to thicken.
- Divide the mix between the 3 glasses and then cover and refrigerate for at least 3 hours.
- Before serving dust each one with come cocoa powder.

Buttermilk Ice Cream Infused With Honey

Ingredients

11/2 cups low-fat evaporated milk

1/2 cup honey

1/4 cup water

2 tsp powdered gelatin

1 1/2 cups buttermilk

Preparation

- Pour the 1/4 cup of water into a jug (heatproof) and add the powdered gelatin. Heat water in a saucepan and then place the jug in the water. Leave it there until the gelatin has completely dissolved.
- Place the evaporated milk in a separate pan and bring to the boil. Remove the heat and carefully stir in the water and gelatin mixture and honey.
- Pour the evaporated milk mixture into a bowl and allow to cool.
- In a separate bowl beat the buttermilk until it is light and fluffy. Now beat the evaporated milk mixture until it becomes frothy, whilst slowly adding the buttermilk.
- Transfer the mixture into a 2L metal container, cover with foil and place in the freezer for at least 3 hours. Remove and blend with an electric mixer until creamy.

Apples - Baked And Stuffed With Mixed Berries

Ingredients

4 apples

2 cups mixed berries (frozen)

4 cardamom pods

2 tsp honey

1/2 cup yoghurt

Preparation

- Place the mixed berries in a sieve and put over a little bowl. Allow to that in the fridge overnight.
- Preheat the oven to 320 deg. F (160 deg. Celsius).
- Remove the cores from the 4 apples, forming a hole in each one that is about 1.5 inches in diameter.
- Using a sharp knife, score around the entire circumference of each apple (aim for the center) and then make a small cut at the bottom where you will then insert a cardamom pod.
- Divide 3/4 of the berries into the apples and before putting them into the over and baking for about 45 minutes, or until apples have softened considerably.
- Place the rest of the berries in a little bowl and mash. Add the yoghurt and honey and stir.

- Serve baked apples topped with yoghurt mixture. Wholesome and delicious!

Frozen Yoghurt Mangoes, Berries, And Passion Fruit

Ingredients

1 medium sized mango

1 cup sliced strawberries

1/4 cup passion fruit pulp

2 cups vanilla yoghurt (low-fat)

Preparation

- Place half of the berries and half of the mango into a blender separately and blend until smooth. Chop the remaining mango and berries and keep separate.

- In a medium sized bowl combine 1/2 cup yoghurt, chopped mango and mango puree. Divide this mixture amongst 8 X 8 ounce (250 ml) disposable cups and place in freezer for 1 hour. Remove once it has become firm.

- Now combine 1/2 cup yoghurt, strawberry puree and remaining sliced strawberries. Distribute the strawberry amongst the 8 cups - on top of mango mixture. Place in freezer for 1 hour and remove once firm.

- Combine the passion fruit pulp and remaining yoghurt. Divide the mixture between the 8 cups and place in freezer once again for an hour. Remove and push an ice cream stick into the center of each cup.

- Cover and freeze again for 3 hours. Remove when ready to serve.

Baked Custard Delight

Ingredients

6 eggs

2/3 Tbsp Stevia powdered extract (1/3 tsp Stevia liquid concentrate)

4 cups hot low-fat milk

1/4 teaspoon ground nutmeg

1 teaspoon vanilla extract

Preparation

- Preheat oven to 320 deg. F (160 deg. Celsius.)
- In large bowl, combine whisked eggs, vanilla extract and Stevia. Slowly stir in hot milk. Pour the custard into a greased oven dish and sprinkle nutmeg on top.
- Pour boiling water into a separate baking dish and put oven dish inside. The water should cover at least 1/2 of the circumference of the oven dish.
- Put in oven and bake for 45 min.

Vanilla Ice-Cream With Berry Topping

Ingredients

1/4 cup custard powder

10 oz. soft tofu

2 tsp vanilla extract

3 cups low fat milk

1 Tbsp Stevia powdered extract (1/2 tsp Stevia liquid concentrate)

Berry Topping

2 1/2 cups mixed berries

2 tsp icing

Preparation

- Pour milk into a saucepan and slowly stir in the custard powder until consistency is smooth. While continuing to stir add the Stevia and milk until the custard starts boiling and thickening. Remove from the heat.
- Place tofu in a blender and blend until smooth.
- Add the vanilla extract and blended tofu to the custard and stir. Allow the mixture to cool before placing in a 14 cm by 21 cm loaf pan. Cover with foil and place in freezer overnight or for at least 3 hours.

- Transfer mixture to 14cm x 21cm (5%-inch x 8Y2-inch) loaf pan. Cover tightly with foil, freeze 3 hours or overnight.
- Remove ice cream from pan and beat with an electric mixer until creamy and smooth. Transfer back to pan, cover and place in freezer for another 3 hours. Repeat the process of beating with electric mixer and freezing twice more.
- To make the berry topping place berries and Stevia in a blender and blend until smooth. Place the finished product in a fine sieve and push through to get rid of all the solid pieces.

Diabetic Chocolate Brownies

Ingredients

2 tbsp unsweetened cocoa powder

4 ½ packets Splenda

4 ½ packets Splenda Granulated Sweetener

16 graham crackers – whole chocolate

2 tsp instant coffee

2 tsp vanilla extract

1/4 tsp salt

2/3 cup diced and pitted dates

2 eggs

1 egg white

1/4 cup semisweet chocolate chips

Preparation

- Preheat oven to 302 deg. F (150 deg. Celsius) and liberally spray cooking spray inside an 8 by 11 1/2 inch baking dish.
- Place graham crackers in food processor and pulse until they turn into crumbs (there should be at least 2 cups worth). Place the crumbs in a bowl, add the cocoa and salt and combine.

- In a large bowl combine the Splenda, egg, egg white and granulated Splenda. Beat with an electric mixer for about 2 min on high until mixture has thickened.
- Next, add coffee granules and vanilla to mixture as well as the chocolate chips, dates and remaining crumbs.
- Transfer the mixture into a baking dish, place in oven, and allow to bake for about 30 minutes. Allow to cool completely before attempting to remove.

Creamy Peach Ice-Cream

Ingredients

2 cups fat-free evaporated milk

1 cup fat-free milk

1/2 cup egg substitute

1/4 teaspoon almond extract

2/3 cup calorie-free sweetener

1 cup diced peaches

Preparation

- Place the evaporated milk, fat-free milk, egg substitute, almond extract and sweeter in a large bowl and beat with and electric mixer until blended. Add diced peaches.
- Transfer blended mix to into freezer container (loaf pan), cover with foil and allow to freeze for at least 3 hours. (Preferably overnight)
- Allow to stand for an hour before serving.

Frozen Bananas Smothered In Nuts

Ingredients

3 large ripe bananas

1/2 cup fat-free vanilla yogurt

½ cup Grape Nuts cereal

Preparation

- Remove peels from bananas and cut each one in half (crosswise)
- Push a wooden stick into the flat end of each banana and then spread vanilla yoghurt all over each one before rolling in the cereal.
- Place bananas on wax paper and allow to freeze for about an hour. Serve frozen.

Great Snack Recipes

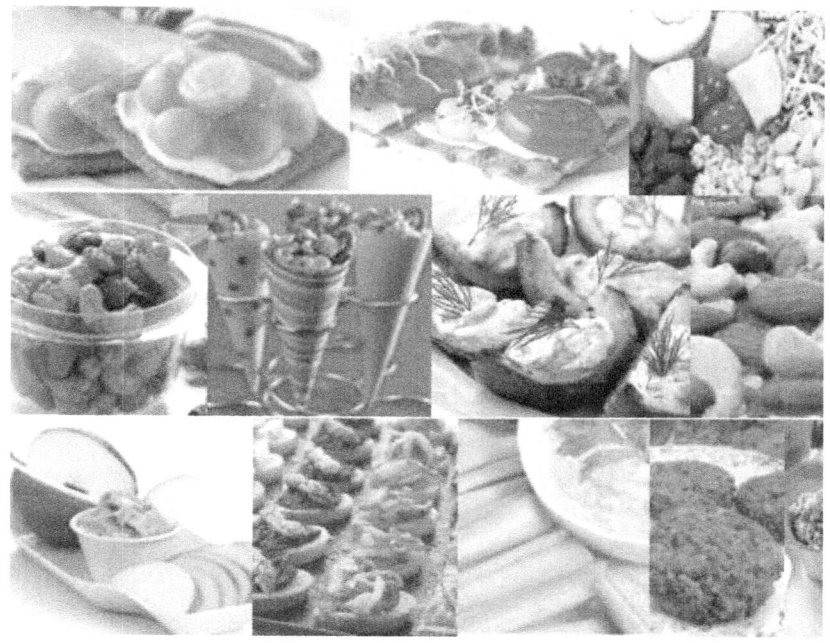

Lemon Biscuits With A Hint Of Lavender

Ingredients

¾ cup all-purpose flour

2 packets Splenda

1 tbsp dried lavender

½ tsp fine sea salt

½ cup almond flour

Zest from one medium sized lemon

2 tbsp honey

2 tbsp arrowroot

½ tsp baking soda

1 chilled stick of unsalted butter (cut into ½ inch pieces)

1 tbsp lemon juice

Preparation

- Preheat oven with oven rack inside to 356 deg. F (180 deg. Celsius)
- Use parchment paper to line a baking sheet.

- Using a food processor combine the flour (almond and all-purpose), Splenda, lavender, baking soda, salt, and arrowroot and pulse.
- Now add the lemon zest and butter and continue to pulse until a coarse meal forms. Add the lemon juice and honey and keep pulsing until a soft dough forms.
- Take the dough and form 1 inch round balls. Press them into discs that are 1 ½ inches in diameter and ¼ inches thick.
- Place the balls on your baking sheet and put in over. Bake for about 10 minutes until they are golden brown.

Delicious Berry Salad

Ingredients

2 tbsp low-fat yoghurt

6 medium sized strawberries (remove stem and cut up)

¼ cup raspberries

¼ cup blueberries

1 tbsp lime juice

1 tbsp mint leaves

1 cup cantaloupe (cubed)

Preparation

- Place all cut up fruit in a medium sized bowl.
- Mix the lime juice, yoghurt, and mint together and then add to the fruit and toss. Serve chilled.

Berry Peach And Apple Salad

Ingredients

1 cup raspberries

1 cup blackberries

1 cup strawberries

1 sliced apples

1 sliced peach

2 cups chopped lettuce

1 tsp crushed almonds

Preparation

Place all ingredients in a large bowl and toss for a refreshing and healthy snack.

Very Berry Popsicle

Ingredients

1 cup black cherries

1 cup blackberries

1 cup water

1/2 tsp ginger

1 cup fat free berry yoghurt

1 cup orange juice (100%, unsweetened)

Preparation

Place all the ingredients in a blender and strain before placing in a popsicle tray and freezing.

Icy Banana And Berry Delight

Ingredients

1 cup strawberries

1 cup blueberries

1/2 banana peeled and sliced

1/2 tsp ginger

1 cup water

1 cup roughly chopped pineapple

Preparation

- Place fruit in medium sized bowl and sprinkle ginger over.
- Toss and then add water. Place ingredients in your popsicle tray and freeze for a chunky icy surprise.

20 More Ideas For Quick And Easy Snacks

We all know what it feels like to get the munchies! It happens without warning and more often than not we end up eating whatever is available. As a diabetic, it is crucial to have healthy snacks on hand and low-carb snacks are your best bet! Here is a list of snacks that won't cause your blood sugar levels to get out of control.

- Hard boiled eggs
- Fresh vegetables with Hummus
- Celery sticks with a peanut butter dip
- Broccoli covered in melted cheese
- Low fat cottage cheese on low-fat whole grain crackers
- Fresh strawberries with low fat yoghurt
- Carrot sticks
- Cucumber slices
- Salad with a low fat dressing
- Snap peas with hummus
- Nuts
- Pickles
- Tomato and mozzarella salad
- Whole grain crackers with sardines and a slice of lemon
- Rye crackers topped with tuna , 2 tsp of light mayonnaise and Dijon mustard to taste
- Tomatoes and mashed avocado on a slice of rye toast.
- Mix of veggies with guacamole
- 1 or 2 dark chocolate squares

- 1 cup sugar-free jelly
- Cheese sandwich – 2 slices whole wheat bread and 1 slice low-fat cheese

Smoothies For Diabetics

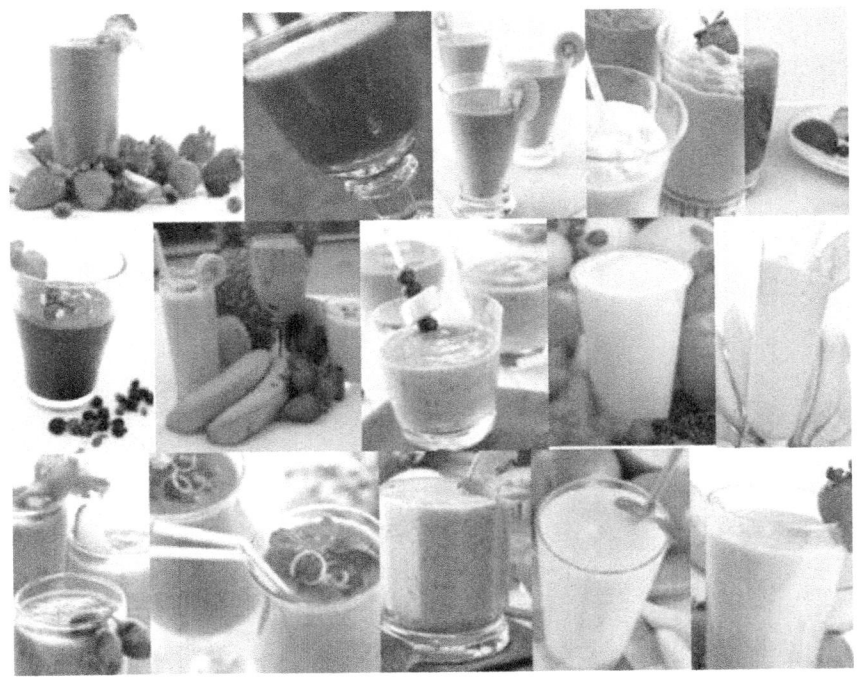

Refreshing Peach Smoothie

Ingredients

2 cups peach slices

1 cup fat-free peach yogurt with no-calorie sweetener

1cup crushed ice or ice cubes

Preparation

Place all ingredients in blender and blend until smooth.

Blueberry Peach Smoothie

Ingredients

2 cups peach slices

½ cup blueberries

1 cup fat free vanilla yoghurt

1 cup crushed ice or ice cubes

Preparation

Place all ingredients in blender and blend until smooth.

Strawberry And Peach Smoothie

Ingredients

2 cups peach slices

½ cup strawberries

1 cup fat free strawberry yoghurt

1 cup crushed ice or ice cubes

Preparation

Place all ingredients in blender and blend until smooth.

Banana Strawberry Smoothie

Ingredients

2 cups diced strawberries

1sliced medium banana

1 cup fat free vanilla yoghurt

1cup ice cubes or crushed ice

1sliced kiwi fruit for garnish

Preparation

In a blender combine all the fruit and yoghurt and blend. Slowly add the ice cubes and continue blending until smooth.

Coffee Vanilla Smoothie

Ingredients

1 cup low fat vanilla yogurt

1/3 cup fat free milk

½ cup ice cubes/crushed ice

1 tsp instant coffee

Preparation

Place all ingredients in blender and blend until smooth.

Strawberry Honey Twist Smoothie

Ingredients

½ medium sized banana, sliced

½ cup fresh strawberries

1 tsp ginger

1/4 cup dry milk powder (non-fat)

1/4 cup apple juice

1 tbsp honey

1 cup ice cubes/crushed ice

Preparation

Place all ingredients in blender and blend until smooth

Almond Blueberry Smoothie

Ingredients

1.5 cups fresh blueberries

1/2 cup fat free Greek yoghurt

2 tbsp wheat germ

2 tbsp skim milk

1/4 cup almonds

2 tsp honey

1 cup ice cubes/crushed ice

Preparation

Place all ingredients in blender and blend until smooth.

Raspberry Peanut Surprise Smoothie

Ingredients

1.5 cups fresh raspberries

2 tbsp skim milk

2 tsp honey

2 tbsp smooth peanut butter

1 cup ice cubes

Preparation

Combine all ingredients in a blender and blend until smooth.

Spinach Apple Smoothie

Ingredients

1 medium sized apple, sliced

2 cups spinach

1/2 cup fat-free Greek Yoghurt

1/3 cup pure apple juice

2 tbsp flax seeds

1 cup ice cubes/crushed ice

1 tsp honey

Preparation

Place all ingredients in blender and blend until smooth.

Cottage Cheese, Raspberry And Cinnamon Smoothie

Ingredients

1.5 cups raspberries

1/2 cup fat free cottage cheese

1 tsp honey

Pinch of cinnamon

2 tbsp rolled oats

1 cup ice cubes/crushed ice

Preparation

Place all ingredients in a blender and blend until smooth.

Blackberry And Honey Smoothie

Ingredients

1.5 cups fresh blackberries

1/2 cup plain fat-free Greek yogurt

2 tsp honey

2 tablespoons almond butter

1 cup ice cubes

Preparation

Place all ingredients in a blender and blend until smooth

Berry And Banana Smoothie

Ingredients

2 cups plain non-fat yogurt

2 bananas, sliced

1 cup fresh strawberries, sliced

1 cup fresh raspberries (alternatively use blueberries or blackberries)

Preparation

Place all ingredients in blender and blend until smooth.

Pineapple And Coconut Smoothie

Ingredients

1 cup fat free or low- fat plain yogurt

1.5 cups fresh pineapple, sliced

1 tsp coconut extract (non-alcoholic)

1 cup ice cubes/crushed ice

Preparation

Place all ingredients in blender and blend until smooth.

Banana And Green Tea Smoothie

Ingredients

1 medium sized banana, sliced

1 cup skim milk

3 tbsp hot water

2 tsps. green tea powder

1 cup crushed ice/ ice cubes

Preparation

- First combine the green tea powder and hot water to form a paste.
- Place all the other ingredients, including the paste into a blender and blend until smooth.

Diabetic Breakfast Smoothie

Ingredients

1/2 cup dry oats (uncooked)

 1 1/2 cups skim milk

1 small banana, sliced

1 tbsp flaxseed

1 tsp coffee extract

Preparation

- Place oats in blender and blend until they become powdery.
- Add the rest of the ingredients and blend until smooth.

Caramel Peanut Smoothie

Ingredients

1 cup unsweetened almond milk

1/2 cup skim milk

2 pkts Splenda

1 tbsp unsweetened cocoa powder

1 tbsp peanut butter

1 tbsp sugar free caramel syrup

1 tbsp ground flax seed

3/4 scoop protein powder (Preferably Vanilla)

Preparation

Place all ingredients in blender and blend until smooth

Strawberry And Cinnamon Smoothie

Ingredients

1 cup fresh strawberries

1/2 cup fat-free vanilla yoghurt

1/2 cup skim milk

3 tbsp flax meal

1/2 tsp cinnamon

Preparation

Place all ingredients in blender and blend until smooth

Banana Mango Smoothie

Ingredients

1 large mango, peeled and sliced

2 medium sized bananas, sliced

2 cup orange juice

2 tbsp maple syrup

1/2 cup plain fat free yogurt

1/8 tsp ground cardamom

Preparation

- Place all ingredients except maple syrup into blender and blend until smooth.
- Slowly add maple syrup to taste.

Supplements

As the incidence of diabetes has risen over the last few years, people have started looking to alternative therapies. Nutritional supplements are highly beneficial to diabetics and have proven to help lower blood sugar levels and to decrease the risk of complications. The nutritional supplements that that I will be discussing are all useful when taken in conjunction with a controlled and healthy diet. In the treatment of diabetes diet should always be the central focus. Nutritional supplements serve to provide the extra nutrients needed by diabetics. Patients who have chosen this path of treatment have seen some great results. It is certainly worth every diabetics while to be informed about the nutritional supplement that have proven to improve insulin function and glucose tolerance.

Here is a list of some of the great supplements that are recommended:

Chromium Picolinate

This is a great supplement for diabetics to take as it helps stabilize blood sugar levels and improve insulin function over time. In the past, patients who have taken up to 1000mcg daily have seen noteworthy improvements in their condition. Interestingly enough a lack of chromium in non diabetics results in diabetic symptoms. It only makes sense that this supplement would improve a diabetic's overall condition.

Vitamin E

Vitamin E supplements help to significantly reduce the incidence of complications in diabetics since it has an anticlotting and anti-inflammatory effect and is a powerful antioxidant. Complications such as coronary heart disease, cataracts and kidney problems are often seen in people who have had diabetes for a long time. Vitamin E can delay or prevent these problems as it helps lower blood fats, improve glucose tolerance, and reduces glycosylation.

Some great natural sources of vitamin E are avocados, nuts and seeds, broccoli, wheatgerm oil, and wholemeal cereals. Eating fresh raw foods and taking supplements is the best way to ensure a sufficient intake of Vitamin E.

Vitamin C

Insulin is instrumental in transporting Vitamin C into the cells of our body. When there is a vitamin C deficiency, complications can arise. Since diabetics naturally struggle with insulin function, they usually have a Vitamin C deficiency, even when their diets are packed with great Vitamin C sources. This deficiency manifests itself in vascular disease, bleeding tendencies, a weakened immune system, poor wound healing, and the degeneration of insulin producing cells in the pancreas.

The RDA for Vitamin C in non-diabetics is approximately 60mg. The general consensus is that those with diabetes should try and take between 120 to 250 mg daily if they are going to see an improvement in their condition and a reduced risk of complications. Diabetics who take this much Vitamin C daily will be able to better maintain their eye health by preventing cataracts and might even reduce the amount of insulin they need over a period of time. Most importantly, their immune systems will be strengthened and their bodies will be better equipped to fight infection. Fruits and vegetables like citrus fruit, mangoes, any green sprouting vegetables, green peppers, guavas, potatoes and berries are great sources of Vitamin C.

Diabetics planning on taking a Vitamin C supplement should first go and get their kidney function tested. This is crucial since too much Vitamin C could prove to be toxic to diabetics who are battling renal insufficiency.

Vitamin B6

You may have heard people refer to the B vitamins as immune boosters. This is because this group of vitamins plays a primary role in the production of antibodies, which are required to fight infection – something which diabetics often struggle with. Not only do these vitamins help diabetics fight infection, but they have also been proven to offer protection against neuropathy. Diabetics who are struggling with any form of peripheral nerve abnormalities should certainly be taking a Vitamin B6 supplement. Vitamin B6 has also been shown to offer significant protection against complications such as coronary heart disease and diabetic retinopathy

Diabetics can benefit greatly from Vitamin B6 supplements. According to Dr. Sarah Brewer "All the B group vitamins are beneficial for people with diabetes as they are involved in the processes which produce energy within body cells." Sources of Vitamin B6 include liver meat, oily fish, bananas, nuts, wholegrains, avocados, egg yolk and green leafy vegetables.

Vitamin B12

Vitamin B12 plays a key role in lowering homocysteine levels. Homocysteine is a naturally occurring amino acid found in blood plasma which can cause complications when its levels within the body are raised. Diabetic retinopathy is one of these complications. Doctors have been treating diabetic retinopathy with Vitamin B12 since the 1950's and the results have been astounding. Diabetics can take up to 2mg a day if necessary. No side effects have been reported, even with such a high dosage.

This vitamin is also helpful in the treatment of diabetic neuropathy and can be found naturally in kidney, meat, sardines, dairy products, eggs, and liver.

Magnesium

Magnesium is an important supplement used by the body in the process of glucose metabolism. Most diabetics have a magnesium deficiency and should consider taking a supplement since it could help prevent both retinopathy and heart disease. Diabetics need up to double the RDA of non-diabetics. This amounts to approximately 600 mg a day.

Magnesium helps maintain a healthy cardiovascular system by decreasing the amount of cholesterol and fat in the blood. It is also helpful in preventing retinopathy and atherosclerosis.

154

Silymarin

Silymarin is a powerful antioxidant found in the herb milk thistle. Studies show that it can help type 2 diabetics by lowering their glucose levels. It also acts as an anti-inflammatory when necessary and has been shown to prevent liver damage and help maintain healthy liver function.

Niacin and Niacinamide

According to Dr. Wright "Niacinamide, one of the B vitamins, is the number one nutrient for treating Type 1 Diabetes." Several experiments done on animals suggest that niacinamide may actually slow down or completely stop the development of Type 1 Diabetes. This is because niacinamide helps slow down the demise of beta cells and plays an important role in glucose tolerance. This naturally reduces the extent of blood vessel and organ damage caused by raised blood sugar levels.

Biotinide

Biotin is part of the B group of vitamins and is used by the body to synthesize and metabolize fatty acids, amino acids, stress hormones, genetic material and glucose. When taken as a supplement by diabetics, Biotin serves to improve insulin sensitivity and most importantly enhance the activity of glucokinase, which is an enzyme used by the liver to process glucose. Studies show that type 1 and 2 diabetics who took this nutrient enjoyed lower blood sugar levels and improved glucose control. Over time some were even able to adjust their insulin requirements.

The recommended dosage of biotin for diabetics is anything between 0.15 mcg and 1mg. Food sources include egg yolks, wholegrains, fish, liver, cauliflower, meat and nuts.

Potassium

All diabetics should be eating a diet that is full of potassium as it is helpful in improving insulin sensitivity, secretion and responsiveness. The incidence of heart disease, atherosclerosis and cancer is reduced in patients who receive a lot of potassium, either through supplementation or diet.

It is preferable for diabetics to receive potassium through their diet as potassium salts can have unpleasant side effects like vomiting, nausea, diarrhea and ulcers. Although most diabetics can handle a lot of potassium, those with kidney failure will not be able to process large amounts and might suffer the consequences of potassium toxicity.

Potassium is found naturally in fresh fruit, seafood, vegetable juices, mushrooms, potatoes, peppers, spinach, lima beans and peas.

Manganese

We all need manganese as it is involved in thyroid hormone function, blood sugar control, and energy metabolism. Diabetics naturally only have half of the manganese found in healthy individuals so they need to be taking manganese supplements. The recommended dosage is 30 mg a day.

Zinc

Zinc has proven to be useful in improving insulin function and in reducing the risk of certain diabetes related complications. Since it plays a crucial role in the storage, synthesis, and secretion of insulin, a deficiency will certainly affect insulin function within the body.

Food sources containing zinc include seafood, offal, wholegrains, eggs, cheese, seafood and brewer's yeast.

Essential Fatty Acids

Both omega-3 and omega-6 have proven to benefit diabetics. Omega-3 helps type 2 diabetics by enhancing insulin secretion and preventing the hardening of arteries. It also reduces vascular complications and insulin resistance. Gamma-linolenic is an omega-6 fatty acid that has proven to help prevent diabetic neuropathy.

Omega-3 oils can be found in pumpkin seeds, soybeans, flaxseed oil, beans, spinach, winter squash, broccoli, cauliflower, as well as mackerel, salmon and cod fish oils. The primary omega-6 oil is called linoleic acid and can be found in peanuts, sesame, corn, safflower, wheatgerm, cottonseed, vegetable and sunflower oils.

Alpha-Lipoic Acid

Alpha-Lipoic acid has successfully been used by doctors to treat adult-onset diabetes for more than 30 years. It is not effective when taken orally so needs to be administered intravenously. A dose of 1,000mg should help to lower insulin resistance and improve the cells ability to use glucose by as much as 55 percent.

Carnitine

There is evidence that Carnitine could play a role in slowing down or even preventing diabetic ketoacidosis. Diabetics who have taken Carnitine supplements also noticed an increase in HDL-cholesterol levels and a decrease in total serum lipid levels.

Vanadium

Vanadium can be found in dill seed, grains, unsaturated vegetable oils and black pepper. Since it mimics insulin, it may improve the diabetics' condition by helping regulate blood sugar. The recommended daily dosage is between 5-2 mg daily. The supplement form to look out for is called Vanadyl Sulfate.

Coenzyme Q10

All human cells contain coenzyme 10, also known as ubiquinone. It helps diabetics in much the same way as Vitamin E does by stimulating insulin production. The recommended dosage is 80 mg a day for approximately 3 months. Diabetics should notice stabilization in their blood sugar levels after this time.

Amino Acids

Diabetics who take amino acid supplements supply their body with some of the raw material needed for the manufacture of insulin, which is made up of 51 amino acids.

Digestive Enzymes

Diabetics have a pancreas that is not functioning as it should. Taking digestive enzymes such as amylase, protease, and lipase will assist diabetics in the absorption and digestion of nutrients.

If you would like to read more about diabetes and get more recipes you can also have a look at my other diabetes book – details below.

Diabetes Diet by John McArthur.

Bibliography

1. Alternative Cures: Bill Gottlieb

2. Alternative Medicine: The Definitive Guide; Second Edition: Larry Trivieri, JR Editor, Introduced by Burton Goldberg.

3. Encyclopedia of Natural Medicine Revised 2nd Edition: Michael Murray N.D. and Joseph Pizzorno N.D.

4. Kilham C 2012. Does America Have a Diabetes Death Wish? Online Article.

5. Natural Approach to Diabetes. Dr. Sarah Brewer, 2005. Piatkus Books Ltd.

6. Newscore 2012. What's the Difference Between Type 1 and Type 2 Diabetes? Online Article

7. Shaw G 2012. How to Avoid – and even reverse – diabetes. Online Article.

More Books By John McArthur

Hypothyroidism
Hypothyroidism: The Hypothyroidism Solution. Hypothyroidism Natural Treatment and Hypothyroidism Diet for Under Active Or Slow Thyroid, Causing Weight Loss Problems, Fatigue, Cardiovascular Disease. John McArthur (Author), Cheri Merz (Editor)

Fibromyalgia And Chronic Fatigue
Fibromyalgia And Chronic Fatigue: A Step-By-Step Guide For Fibromyalgia Treatment And Chronic Fatigue Syndrome Treatment. Includes Fibromyalgia Diet And Chronic Fatigue Diet And Lifestyle Guidelines. John McArthur (Author), Cheri Merz (Editor)

Yeast Infection
Candida Albicans: Yeast Infection Treatment. Treat Yeast Infections With This Home Remedy. The Yeast Infection Cure. John McArthur (Author)

Heart Disease
Hypertension - High Blood Pressure: How To Lower Blood Pressure Permanently In 8 Weeks Or Less, The Hypertension Treatment, Diet and Solution. John McArthur (Author)

Cholesterol Myth: Lower Cholesterol Won't Stop Heart Disease. Healthy Cholesterol Will. Cholesterol Recipe Book & Cholesterol Diet. Lower Cholesterol Naturally Keep Cholesterol Healthy. John McArthur (Author), Cheri Merz (Editor)

Heart Disease Prevention and Reversal: How To Prevent, Cure and Reverse Heart Disease Naturally For A Healthy Heart. John McArthur (Author)

Diabetes

Diabetes Diet: Diabetes Management Options. Includes a Diabetes Diet Plan with Diabetic Meals and Natural Diabetes Food, Herbs and Supplements for Total Diabetes Control. Delicious Recipes. John McArthur (Author), Corinne Watson (Editor)

Diabetes Cooking: 93 Diabetes Recipes for Breakfast, Lunch, Dinner, Snacks and Smoothies. A Guide to Diabetes Foods to Help You Prepare Healthy Delicious ... Diabetic Meals and Natural Diabetes Food) John McArthur (Author), Corinne Watson (Editor)

Stress and Anxiety

From Stressful to Successful in 4 Easy Steps: Stress at Work? Stress in Relationship? Be Stress Free. End Stress and Anxiety. Excellent Stress Management, Stress Control and Stress Relief Techniques. John McArthur (Author)

Anxiety and Panic Attacks: Anxiety Management. Anxiety Relief. The Natural And Drug Free Relief For Anxiety Attacks, Panic Attacks And Panic Disorder. John McArthur (Author), Cheri Merz (Editor)

Back and Neck Pain

The 15 Minute Back Pain and Neck Pain Management Program: Back Pain and Neck Pain Treatment and Relief 15 Minutes a Day No Surgery No Drugs. Effective, Quick and Lasting Back and Neck Pain Relief. John

McArthur (Author)

Arthritis

Arthritis: Arthritis Relief for Osteoarthritis, Rheumatoid Arthritis, Gout, Psoriatic Arthritis, and Juvenile Arthritis. Follow The Arthritis Diet, Cure and Treatment Free Yourself From The Pain. John McArthur (Author)

Depression

How to Break the Grip of Depression: Read How Robert Declared War On Depression ... And Beat It! John McArthur (Author)

Pregnancy

Pregnancy Nutrition: Pregnancy Food. Pregnancy Recipes. Healthy Pregnancy Diet. Pregnancy Health. Pregnancy Eating and Recipes. Nutritional Tips and 63 Delicious Recipes for Moms-to-Be. Corinne Watson (Author), John McArthur (Author)

Pregnancy and Childbirth: Expecting a Baby. Pregnancy Guide. Pregnancy What to Expect. Pregnancy Health. Pregnancy Eating and Recipes. Cheri Merz (Author), John McArthur (Author)

Allergies

Allergy Free: Fast Effective Drug-free Relief for Allergies. Allergy Diet. Allergy Treatments. Allergy Remedies. Natural Allergy Relief. John McArthur (Author), Cheri Merz (Editor)

Made in the USA
Coppell, TX
21 March 2020

17450628R00095